C000044250

LITTLE BOOK OF
MOUSTACHES

Rufus Cavendish

THE LITTLE BOOK OF MOUSTACHES

Copyright © Summersdale Publishers Limited, 2013

Research by Abi McMahon

Page design by Stephen Wildish

Summersdale Publishers Ltd
46 West Street
Chichester
West Sussex
PO19 1RP
UK

www.summersdale.com

Printed and bound in the Czech Republic

ISBN: 978-1-84953-490-1

Substantial discounts on bulk quantities of Summersdale books are available to corporations, professional associations and other organisations. For details contact Nicky Douglas by telephone: +44 (0) 1243 756902, fax: +44 (0) 1243 786300 or email: nicky@summersdale.com.

Contents

The How-Tos and Wherewithals of Successful Moustache Growing

While the only thing required to grow a moustache is the passage of time and some appropriately placed hair follicles, honing that moustache into a fine facial accessory requires some particular knowledge, skill and equipment. Here are some crucial tips and tools to ensure you don't half-tache anything.

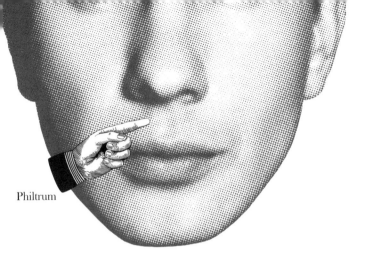

Philtrum

ANATOMY OF A MOUSTACHE

Philtrum: The elegantly creased bit between your upper lip and your nose. While some styles cover your upper lip in its entirety, others require shaving in the middle; in these cases the philtrum acts as a tiny centre parting.

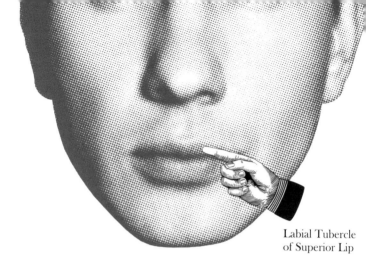

Labial Tubercle
of Superior Lip

Labial Tubercle of Superior Lip:
Henceforth known as your 'top lip'. Certain
fashions of moustache will trespass into this
area, causing food to become trapped in their
tendrils. As any experienced moustachio
knows, this gives the very great benefit of never
having to pack lunch again.

TACHE TOOLS

Moustache Wax
It simply wouldn't be possible to execute a dashing moustache twirl without the appropriate moustache wax. Any curled, crimped or crazy tache requires a healthy dollop of moustache wax to help it keep its shape.

Razor
Although wielding a straight razor gives one a dashing 'Sweeney Todd' air, the modern moustachio can achieve any style with today's safer razors. Different numbers of blades will affect accuracy; use a single-blade razor for delicate work and multi-blades for the bulk shave.

Moustache Trimmer

A trimmer is a moustache-have for neat, well-to-do taches. Perfect for maintaining a regular length, though not suited to handling the longer styles, the electric trimmer is even available with batteries, for when one is on the tache dash.

Comb

As facial hair rarely knows what's best for it, a comb is essential for styling your tache. The ideal comb has a handle, is made of strong enough material that it can subdue stubborn, wiry hair, but also possesses short, finely spaced teeth for intricate styling. For the thinner, more delicate moustache an especially fine-toothed comb may be required.

Scissors

When it's time to trim the longer tache, your best tool is a pair of good stainless steel scissors with sharp, straight blades. Wield the blades freestyle when attending to the truly long hairs, and pair with a comb for smart, fulsome facial fuzz.

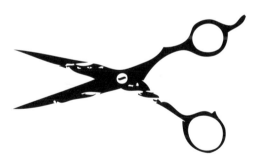

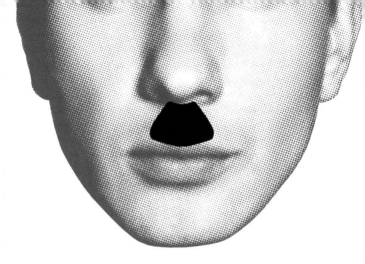

The

CHAPLIN

NEVER BEFORE HAS FACIAL HAIR SUFFERED SUCH A HEADY RISE AND PLUMMETING FALL.

THIS TIDDLY TOOTHBRUSH TACHE
IS FOR OLD-SCHOOL COMEDY FANS
ONLY. IT MAY SIT UNDER YOUR
NOSE LIKE HAIRY BUCK TEETH,
BUT YOU'RE REALLY CARRYING A
LITTLE SLICE OF HISTORY UPON
YOUR PHILTRUM.

Grow

DIFFICULTY: 🥸 🥸

1 Grow the hair on your upper lip to full length with no parting, without trimming the length.

2 Shave either side of the moustache, leaving a 3–5 cm strip in the centre.

3 When maintaining the shape of the Chaplin, taper the sides out slightly to avoid a regimented, vertical effect. It is not necessary to use wax on the hair, as it should give the wearer an endearingly unkempt appearance.

4 Learn mad tricks with your bowler hat in order to show off your Chaplin at its best.

Make

DIFFICULTY: 🥸 🥸 🥸

REQUIRED: THIN ELASTIC, METAL SKEWER, THICK CARDBOARD, FAKE FUR, TAPE MEASURE, GLUE

1 Cut the shape of a toothbrush moustache from the thick cardboard, ensuring the top is no bigger than the width of your nostrils and the base no wider than 5 cm.

2 Measure your head from ear to ear and cut the elastic a little shorter, to allow it to stretch.

3 Punch a hole either side of the cardboard tache and firmly tie the elastic, trimming the excess.

4 Cut the fake fur to the shape of the toothbrush moustache and glue on.

5 If strangers approach you with spare change, you have taken the 'lovable tramp' look too far.

Sport the Chaplin when taking
elegant pratfalls.

Simply must be paired with bowler, cane
and ill-fitting trousers for best effect.

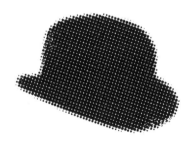

HUMANS HAVE BEEN
SHAPING THEIR HAIR
SINCE NEOLITHIC TIMES;
THE EARLIEST SHAVING
RAZORS DISCOVERED DATE
BACK TO 30,000 YEARS
AGO AND TAKE THE FORM
OF FLINT BLADES.

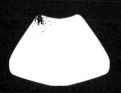

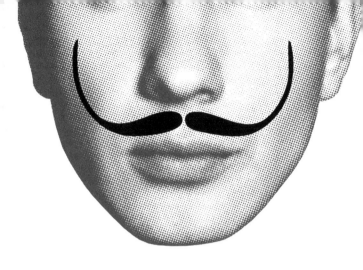

The

DALÍ

WHY WEAR YOUR MOUSTACHE THE RIGHT WAY UP WHEN YOU COULD WEAR IT UPSIDE DOWN?

SALVADOR DALÍ,
THE SURREALIST ARTIST,
BROUGHT ART TO LIFE WITH HIS
UNUSUAL MOUSTACHE THRUSTING
OFF HIS FACE AT A 45° ANGLE. THIS
IS THE TACHE THAT SAYS 'I'M
HERE AND SO ARE THE LOBSTERS.'

Grow

DIFFICULTY: 🥸 🥸 🥸 🥸 🥸

REQUIRED: A SINGLE BLADE, MOUSTACHE WAX

1 Using a single blade, trim your moustache horizontally until it is a sliver, with no parting.

2 Keeping the shape, grow the hair long, especially at the tips. A full Dalí can take upwards of six months, so patience is required.

3 Finally, work a generous amount of wax into the moustache, beginning in the middle and working outwards to the tips – enough so that it will hold when you shape it upwards towards your eyebrows.

4 Can be worn either straight or with an inward curl, the Dalí defies arbitrary restrictions on reality.

Make

DIFFICULTY: 🥸

REQUIRED: THICK PIPE CLEANERS,
THEATRICAL GLUE, RULER

1 Bend a pipe cleaner in half and twist the two halves tightly together.

2 Measure a couple of centimetres from the end of the pipe cleaner, this will be the section that attaches to your lip.

3 Pinch the pipe cleaner into a tight upward bend for your tache prong. Repeat for the other side of the tache.

4 Dab a little glue onto the pipe cleaners and fasten to either side of your top lip. Twitch wildly upon spying something surreal.

Partner your Dalí with your long cape, your bespoke walking stick and your pet ocelot.

Lightly touch your Dalí to indicate that you have enjoyed any visual pun you espy.

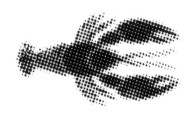

SINCE I DON'T SMOKE, I DECIDED TO GROW A MOUSTACHE – IT IS BETTER FOR THE HEALTH.

SALVADOR DALÍ

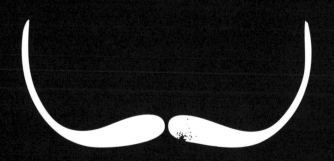

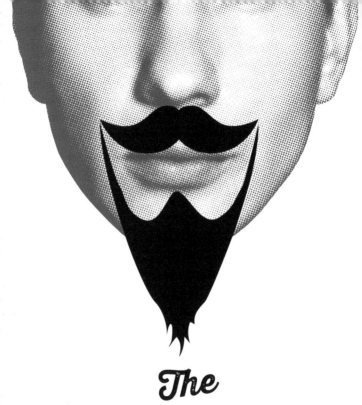

The

FAWKES

REMEMBER, REMEMBER, THE 5TH OF NOVEMBER, FOR GUNPOWDER, TREASON AND TACHE.

RECENTLY RECLAIMED BY THE INTERNET, THE FAWKES MAY NOT BE THE ONLY REVOLUTIONARY FACIAL HAIR BUT IT'S CERTAINLY THE POINTIEST.

Grow

DIFFICULTY:

1 The starting point for the Fawkes is a moustache of regular length, and a tapered goatee with the hair trimmed to a point.

2 Using the corner of a razor, shave a parting on your philtrum, slanting the edges of your tache inwards. Use wax to shape the tips of your moustache until they are pointing upwards.

3 Your goatee should start below the tips of your moustache, with an isolated strip of hair leading downwards from your bottom lip. To create the strip, hold your razor with the blade vertical and shave outward in brief strokes, ensuring the hair either side of the bare skin remains intact.

4 This Fawkes is perfect for all occasions with the exception of Bonfire Night, on which you may be put on the bonfire.

Make

DIFFICULTY: 🥸 🥸 🥸 🥸 🥸

REQUIRED: FELT, SCISSORS, PINS, NEEDLE, THREAD, SEWING MACHINE (OPTIONAL), PAPER, PEN, RIBBON

1 Draw two templates on the paper, one for the moustache and another for the beard. Ensure the beard template reaches your ears and has two points that will sit either side of your mouth, to fasten the moustache to.

2 Pin the templates to the felt and cut around them.

3 Either by hand, or using a sewing machine, sew around the edges of the felt shapes for a decorative effect. Sew a length of ribbon to the ends of the beard shape, long enough to tie around your head.

4 Pin the moustache to the points of the beard and sew the two shapes together to complete the Fawkes.

(Traditional) Partner your Fawkes with the latest lace ruff, buckled hat and doublet.

(Modern) A simple black suit and white shirt will ensure you don't suffer the worst of fashion punishments: being laughed at on the Internet.

Perfect for making an explosive entry to soirées and The State Opening of Parliament.

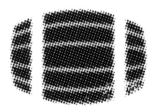

THE WORLD RECORD FOR THE LONGEST MOUSTACHE IS HELD BY RAM SINGH CHAUHAN OF INDIA, AT 14 FT LONG.

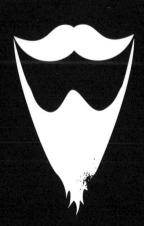

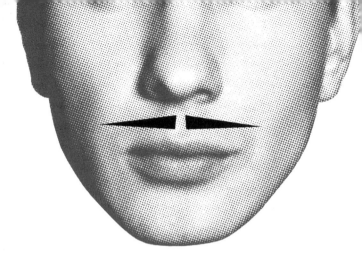

The

GABLE

THE GABLE MUST BE WORN
WITH EXTREME CAUTION, AS IT
CONTAINS ENOUGH SEDUCTIVE
ENERGY TO POWER THREE
CITIES.

NEATLY PARTED AND TRIMMED,
THIS MOUSTACHE MUST SIT ON
YOUR UPPER LIP WITH ALL THE
CONFIDENCE-CUM-ARROGANCE OF A
HOLLYWOOD LEADING MAN.

Grow

DIFFICULTY: 🥸 🥸

1 Clip your moustache to a short, tight length, not more than a few millimetres. This can also be done using scissors.

2 The Gable is a classic pencil moustache – shave down from your natural tache hairline to flatten the taper to a straight line. Shave down below the tache to create the ultra-thin shape.

3 Holding the razor so the blade is vertical, shave across your philtrum in short, sharp strokes to divide the moustache.

4 Wreak devastation on the hearts and knees of any leading lady... or leading man.

Make

DIFFICULTY: 🥸 🥸

REQUIRED: SAUCEPAN, GLASS BOWL, MIXING SPOON, 125 g CHOCOLATE, PIPING BAG, GREASEPROOF PAPER

1 Break the chocolate into small pieces and place into the glass bowl.

2 Place the bowl over a saucepan halfway full with boiling water and let the chocolate melt. Stir to ensure the chocolate is fully melted.

3 Let the melted chocolate cool for a few minutes before filling the piping bag.

4 Pipe thin, wide-set 'v' shapes onto the greaseproof paper.

5 Serve with coffee and your best lines.

The important thing isn't what you put on when you wear the Gable, but what others take off.

Don the Gable when you wish to indicate that frankly, you don't give a damn.

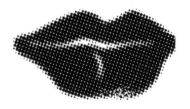

BEING KISSED BY A MAN WHO DIDN'T WAX HIS MOUSTACHE WAS LIKE EATING AN EGG WITHOUT SALT.

RUDYARD KIPLING

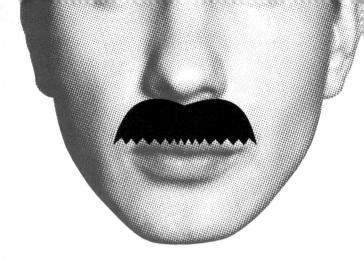

The

GROUCHO

GROUCHO MARX STARTED EXAGGERATING HIS MOUSTACHE EARLY IN HIS VAUDEVILLE DAYS, UNWITTINGLY CREATING THE FACE THAT LAUNCHED A THOUSAND NOVELTY DISGUISES.

AN EYE-CATCHING THICK BLACK RECTANGLE, THIS MOUSTACHE ALMOST SHOOTS QUICK-FIRE WIT BY ITSELF.

Grow

DIFFICULTY:

1. Grow the hair on your upper lip until it is roughly half a centimetre wider than your mouth on either side.

2. Shape the sides so that it is squared off rather than tapered.

3. Maintain a regular length by trimming the hair to the same length across the whole.

4. Walk bent forward at a right angle to show your new Groucho to the best effect.

Make

DIFFICULTY:
REQUIRED: BLACK GREASEPAINT, RAG OR CLOTH

1 Dip the rag in the greasepaint and smear a thick rectangle across your upper lip.

2 Extend the rectangle to slightly beyond your mouth either side.

3 Optional: paint thick eyebrows to have the lip carpet match the drapes.

4 Casually insult your guests; with the Groucho they will mistake your abuse for witty, good humour.

Your Groucho is best enjoyed while
smoking an exploding cigar.

Employ your Groucho when
you wish to stand out from your
comedy-troupe siblings.

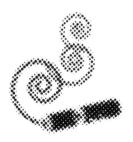

'THERE'S A MAN OUTSIDE
WITH A BIG BLACK
MOUSTACHE.'

'TELL HIM I'VE GOT ONE.'

GROUCHO MARX

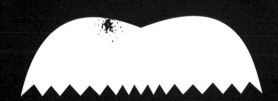

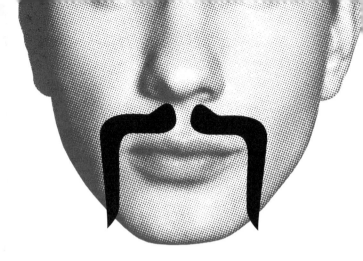

The

HOGAN

AS SQUARE AS WEARER
HULK HOGAN'S JAW, THIS
IS A TACHE THAT BESTOWS
UPON ITS OWNER PLENTY
OF ATTITUDE (DISCLAIMER:
ACTUAL FIGHTING ABILITY NOT
GUARANTEED).

STILL, EVERYONE WILL BE FAR TOO
IN AWE OF YOUR FACIAL HAIR TO
WANT TO TEST THAT.

Grow

DIFFICULTY:

1 The Hogan is a horseshoe moustache and its eventual shape should reflect this. There is no upper lip maintenance required, but some trimming necessary on the 'branches' for shape.

2 Once your facial hair is medium length, shave your jaw and chin, creating facial furniture that reaches down the sides of the mouth to your jawline.

3 That's it! Growing the Hogan requires no skill at all, just like wrestling!

4 The older grower may experience a 'badger' effect. Fear not, this only increases the potency of the Hogan.

Make

DIFFICULTY:

REQUIRED: PLAIN BANDANA, SPONGE, BLACK FABRIC PAINT

1 Cut the sponge into a square-ish horseshoe shape.

2 Fold the bandana by taking a corner and bringing it to its diagonal opposite, to create a triangle.

3 Coat one side of the sponge in fabric paint, ensuring it is fully covered but not dripping.

4 With the bandana lying flat on a hard surface, print the moustache in the centre of the longest side, firmly and without smudging.

5 Once dry, tie the bandana around your face and look like a total badass.

Wear your Hogan with a gaudy bandana
and a few scraps of spandex.

Smooth your Hogan after wrestling your
opponent to inevitable defeat.

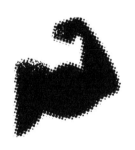

IN 2004 INDIAN POLICE
OFFICERS WERE OFFERED A
PAY RISE IF THEY GREW A
MOUSTACHE, IN THE BELIEF
THAT IT HELPED THEM
COMMAND MORE RESPECT.

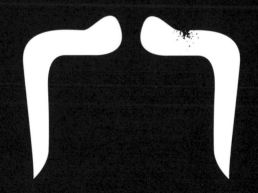

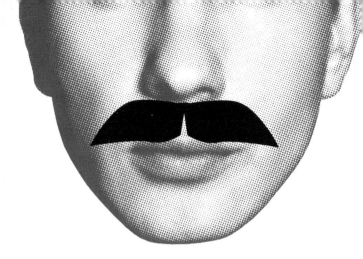

The

MAGNUM
P.I.

TOM SELLECK, ALREADY PURE MASCULINITY FROM HEAD TO FOOT, DISTILLED THE GOOD STUFF FOR HIS TACHE.

VERIFIED AS 99.9-PER-CENT-PROOF TESTOSTERONE, THIS MOUSTACHE COULD FIGHT CRIME ALL BY ITSELF – IT JUST NEEDS SOMEONE TO TRANSPORT IT FROM CRIME SCENE TO CRIME SCENE.

Grow

DIFFICULTY: 🥸 🥸

1. Grow a full upper lip of hair, allowing the length to cover your top lip.

2. Keeping the hair long, trim with scissors for a neat appearance.

3. Using a comb, but no wax, direct the hairs outward, creating a slight parting in the middle.

4. Hop in your Ferrari and cruise for crime.

Make

DIFFICULTY: 🥸 🥸 🥸 🥸
REQUIRED: READY-MADE CHOCOLATE BISCUIT MIX, GREASEPROOF PAPER, KNIFE, ROLLING PIN, BAKING TRAY

1 Add butter and water to the biscuit mix and chill in the fridge for an hour.

2 Roll the mix on a lightly floured surface until roughly half a centimetre thick.

3 Draw the Magnum P. I. tache on greaseproof paper and cut out. Spread your template flat on your biscuit mix and cut around it with a sharp knife.

4 Carefully place the biscuit moustaches on a greased baking tray, ensuring they are not touching. Cook for 20 minutes at 180°C.

5 Leave to cool. Wear (or eat!) while lounging on the beach.

Aviators? Check. Baseball cap? Check.
Hawaiian shirt? Check. You may
don your tache.

The masculinity of your Selleck must be
reflected in the density of your chest hair.

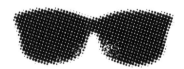

HE THAT HATH A BEARD IS MORE THAN A YOUTH, AND HE THAT HATH NO BEARD IS LESS THAN A MAN.

WILLIAM SHAKESPEARE

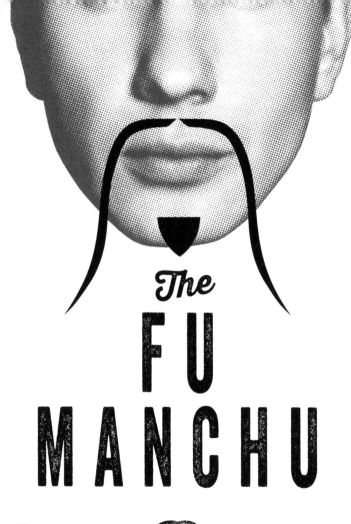

The FU MANCHU

A FORERUNNER IN THE MOUSTACHE SUBCATEGORY 'VILLAINOUS FACIAL HAIR', IF YOU BEAR A FU MANCHU MOUSTACHE, YOU ARE ALMOST DEFINITELY A MASTER CRIMINAL.

THE LONG, THIN MOUSTACHE OF SAX ROHMER'S FICTIONAL CRIMINAL GENIUS FU MANCHU, THIS IS A MUST-WEAR WHEN YOU WANT EVIL TO LITERALLY DRIP FROM YOUR FACE.

Grow

DIFFICULTY:

1 Grow your tache past the corners of your mouth, trimming the length to between 3–5 mm and shave a division at your philtrum.

2 The moustache should sit between your lip and your nose without touching either body part. To achieve this, shave a thin strip above your lip, no more than a few millimetres wide.

3 Do not trim the ends of your moustache, but let the hair grow so it is long and hanging off the face. This can be grown to any length between an inch and passing your chin. As with the Dalí, a good length can take upwards of six months.

4 Hatch a diabolical plan.

Make

DIFFICULTY: 〜〜 〜〜 〜〜 〜〜 〜〜

REQUIRED: 8 g SQUID INK, 1 TSP WATER,
400 g PASTA FLOUR, 200 g SEMOLINA,
4 LARGE EGGS, 3 LARGE EGG YOLKS

1 Make a paste with the squid ink and water.

2 Mix the flour and semolina, make a well and add the paste, eggs and yolks. Press into a crumbly dough then place onto a clean surface and knead for 5 minutes.

3 Divide into four or five portions. Roll each portion flat and fold over itself, repeating the process until the texture is smooth. Roll for a last time to the thickness you require.

4 Cut into long, thin strips. Cook fresh by boiling for 2–3 minutes. Hang pasta from your lip and raise an assassin army.

The Fu Manchu is perfect for inspiring fear and awe in your army of assassins.

It is a truth universally acknowledged that any man in possession of the Fu Manchu must be in need of an equally dastardly nemesis.

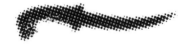

THE OLDEST KNOWN PORTRAIT OF A MOUSTACHE DATES BACK TO 300 BC AND PORTRAYS A SCYTHIAN HORSEMAN.

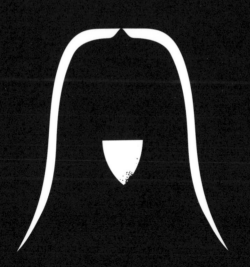

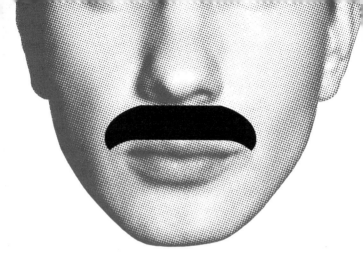

The

MERCURY

QUEEN ARE RUMOURED TO HAVE INVENTED THE MUSIC VIDEO PURELY TO ALLOW THE WORLD TO SEE FRONTMAN FREDDIE MERCURY'S MOUSTACHE.

MORE SONG-STRAINER THAN SOUP-STRAINER, THIS HEAVY MOUSTACHE WILL FILTER YOUR DULCET TONES BETTER THAN ANY AUTO-TUNE.

DIFFICULTY:

1 Your starter tache should be roughly 1 cm wider than your mouth.

2 Keeping the base of your oral ornament straight, use a razor to shape the top into a slight downward curve.

3 Using clippers, trim until the hair is full but not bristly.

4 Throw an outrageously decadent party in celebration of your moustache.

Make

DIFFICULTY: 🥸 🥸 🥸

REQUIRED: THICK MATERIAL OF YOUR CHOICE,
SCISSORS, NEEDLE, YARN, PINS,
METAL KEY RING

1 Fold your material in half – felt or fake leather is a
good choice for this craft – and pin your tachetastic
template to the centre.

2 Cut around the template, resulting in two
moustache shapes. From the same material cut a
narrow strip long enough to be folded over.

3 Pin your two moustaches together and sew at the
edges using a blanket stitch, leaving a gap near one
of the ends wide enough for the strip of material.

4 Fold the strip through the centre of the key ring
and insert the ends into the gap in the moustache,
sewing shut with back stitch. This can be used to attach to
your keys.

The Mercury will increase the wearer's range by an octave.*

To appear at your most virile, pair your Mercury with a plunging vest, tight, white trousers and an abundant chest rug.

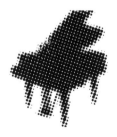

*Validity of this claim cannot be guaranteed.

WONDERFULLY POWERFUL EFFECT UPON A MAN'S WHOLE EXPRESSION. THE IDEA OF VIRILITY, SPIRIT AND MANLINESS THAT IT CONVEYS IS SO GREAT THAT IT WAS A LONG TIME THE SPECIAL PRIVILEGE OF OFFICERS OF THE ARMY TO WEAR IT.

MRS. C. E. HUMPHRY, FROM
ETIQUETTE FOR EVERY DAY

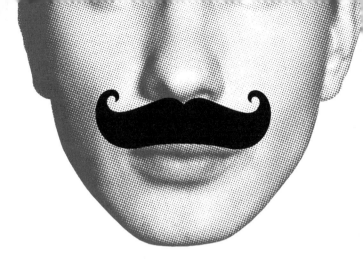

The
NIETZSCHE

NIETZSCHE'S MOUSTACHE ONCE ALLEGEDLY SAID, 'THE CLEAN-SHAVEN LIP IS DEAD', A PHILOSOPHICAL STATEMENT THAT HAS RUNG TRUE WITH MOUSTACHE-WEARERS AND NIHILISTS THROUGH THE AGES.

THIS LARGE HANDLEBAR MOUSTACHE MAKES AS PROFOUND A STATEMENT AT HIPSTER PARTIES AS ANY OF HIS PHILOSOPHIES.

Grow

DIFFICULTY:

1 This is a hefty handlebar, and should extend beyond the wearer's face. The hair should be grown long and full, reaching over the wearer's top lip.

2 As the hair grows, comb once a day to create a split and direct the hairs.

3 After at least three weeks, curl the ends of your tache around your finger or a pencil and wax into position.

4 There is no need to trim this tache – the longer it is, the more wisdom it contains!

Make

DIFFICULTY: 〜 〜 〜 〜 〜

REQUIRED: FELTING NEEDLE, RAW WOOL, YARN, CARDBOARD, HAIRSPRAY, GLUE

1 Ensure your wool is slightly longer and thicker than you would like your final facial furniture to be and tie yarn tightly round the centre, trimming and tucking the edges into the wool.

2 Using a felting needle, stab sharply up and down until the wool is compacted and bonded together. Cover the yarn with a small amount of wool and repeat.

3 Cut a slightly smaller tache from the cardboard and glue to the wool, pressing down firmly.

4 Spray the wool with hairspray and twirl the ends up into a handlebar.

5 Raise to the face to greatly increase how intelligent you look.

As the person with the largest moustache is invariably the most intelligent, the Nietzsche is essential for academic success.

The Nietzsche is perennially fashionable with radicals, free-thinkers and hipsters.

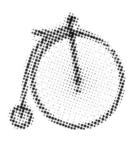

SOME VICTORIAN MEN OVERCAME THE CHALLENGE OF EATING SOUP WHILE IN POSSESSION OF A MOUSTACHE BY USING A SPOON WITH A BUILT-IN MOUSTACHE PROTECTOR.

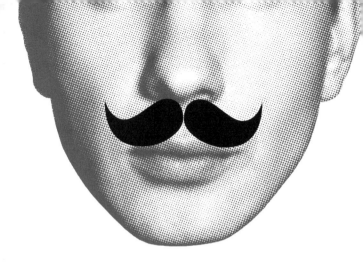

The

POIROT

A PRECISE, FUSSY MOUSTACHE FOR A PRECISE, FUSSY MAN. POIROT, AGATHA CHRISTIE'S FAMOUS FICTIONAL BELGIAN DETECTIVE, WAS AS CAREFUL IN GROOMING HIS TIGHTLY UPTURNED TACHE AS HE WAS IN INVESTIGATING CRIME SCENES.

THIS IS A MOUSTACHE THAT ASKS FOR AN ALIBI IN THE POLITEST OF TERMS.

Grow

DIFFICULTY:

1 Shave your tache so that it is shorter than the width of your mouth and curves down to the tips.

2 Keeping the centre trimmed short, grow the hair until it is long enough to shape into an upward curl.

3 Using a generous amount of wax, shape your tache, ensuring it is stuck firmly to your face.

4 Solve mysteries, such as where you last left your keys.

Make

DIFFICULTY: 🥸 🥸 🥸

REQUIRED: BLACK POLYMER CLAY, ROLLING
PIN, SHARP KNIFE, TOOTHPICK,
OVEN TRAY, GREASEPROOF PAPER,
NECKLACE CHAIN

1 Roll out the clay to roughly 2 mm thickness and
trace the shape of the Poirot with the toothpick.

2 Cut out the moustache using a sharp knife and,
with the toothpick, press a hole in the centre of
each point, not too close to the edge.

3 Line the oven tray with greaseproof paper and bake
at 110°C for 30 minutes.

4 Allow to cool, then fasten to the chain by prising
open a link at each end and hooking through the
holes, before clamping it closed again. Raise to your
mouth when you spy a clue.

Warning: wearing the Poirot attracts an unusual amount of crime in the vicinity, which you will be expected to solve.

The deerstalker and pipe is so passé. Pair your Poirot with matching bow tie and waistcoat to be the ultimate dapper detective.

The well-turned-out detective must wear a protective moustache-net in bed each night, to protect the hard-won curl.

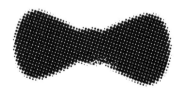

AROUND 50 TOURISTS VISIT ISTANBUL EVERY DAY TO RECEIVE MOUSTACHE AND BEARD IMPLANTS. IN MANY CULTURES A HEALTHY MOUSTACHE IS A SIGN OF HEALTH AND VIRILITY.

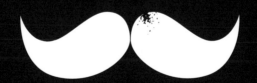

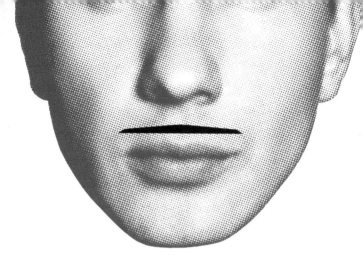

The
WATERS

IF YOUR MAIN HOBBIES INVOLVE LOOMING, WEARING NARROW SUITS AND THOROUGHLY DISCONCERTING MAIDEN AUNTS, WATERS' LIP-SKIMMING PENCIL MOUSTACHE IS FOR YOU.

JOHN WATERS' MOUSTACHE IS NEARLY AS TRANSGRESSIVE AS THE FILMS HE MAKES AND SHOULD BE ADOPTED IF YOU WOULD LIKE A CULT FOLLOWING, OR INDEED A CULT.

Grow

DIFFICULTY: ~ ~

1 Shave your moustache to exactly the length of your lip.

2 Using short, careful strokes, shave from the top of your tache down, until all that remains is a thin line, with no gap between hair and lip.

3 Trim the hair to its shortest possible length without reducing to stubble.

4 See also: Gomez Addams.

Make

DIFFICULTY: 🥸 🥸 🥸

REQUIRED: FLESH-COLOURED ELASTICISED MATERIAL, SCISSORS, NEEDLE, FLESH-COLOURED THREAD, THICK YARN (COLOUR TO SUIT YOUR PERSONAL CHOICE), PINS, TAPE MEASURE

1 Measure the length of your forefinger, and the circumference of its base, and cut your material slightly larger than that.

2 Overlap the longest edges to create a tube and pin in shape. Use the thread to sew together and hem the ends using a zigzag stitch.

3 Using thick yarn, stitch over the join in tightly packed stitches to create a solid, thin line running the length of the tube.

4 Dress your finger in its tache suit to be the first in loveable creep fashion.

Wear the Waters when you wish to disconcert passers-by and strangers, and perhaps even friends and family.

The Waters is essential dress when challenging taboos and people's gross-out levels.

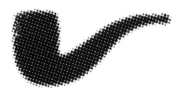

THE WORLD BEARD
AND MOUSTACHE
CHAMPIONSHIPS TAKE
PLACE EVERY YEAR.
THEY RECOGNISE
EIGHT CATEGORIES OF
MOUSTACHE; NATURAL,
ENGLISH, DALI, HANDLEBAR,
WILD WEST, FU MANCHU,
IMPERIAL AND FREESTYLE.

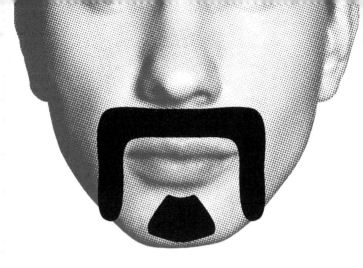

The

ZAPPA

ZAPPA ROCKED HIS FACIAL HAIR NEARLY AS HARD AS HE ROCKED THE STAGE.

DABBLING IN THE DUAL GENRES OF THE MOUSTACHE AND THE SOUL PATCH, THE ZAPPA COMES AS STANDARD WITH WILD, CURLY HAIR AND A SYNCLAVIER, A MUST-HAVE FOR THE MODERN-DAY ECCENTRIC GENIUS ABOUT TOWN.

Grow

DIFFICULTY: 🥸 🥸 🥸

1 Shave your moustache so that it extends around the upper lip and down towards your chin, exceeding your mouth by roughly 5 cm.

2 Grow a rectangular patch of hair originating from the centre of your bottom lip but not reaching your jaw, creating a large soul patch.

3 Trim the hair to an even length, but not too short, as the ends of the tache should droop slightly.

4 Master a new music genre. Again.

Make

DIFFICULTY: 🥸 🥸

REQUIRED: PLAIN WHITE MUG,
CERAMIC PAINT PEN

1 Starting 2 cm below the rim of the mug, draw the outline of your Zappa.

2 The soul patch should sit centred to the moustache, starting just above the bottom points of the tache. It should be a wide rectangle.

3 Fill the outline of your tache and soul patch and leave to dry.

4 Hold mug to lips and drink pure talent, twice a day.

Wear your Zappa when defying both mainstream political thought and society's belief that you *can* have too much synclavier music.

Impress your friends with your love of orchestral and popular music, preferably both at the same time.

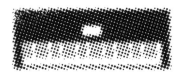

THE AVERAGE MOUSTACHE TRAPS ROUGHLY A PINT AND A HALF OF BEER A YEAR.

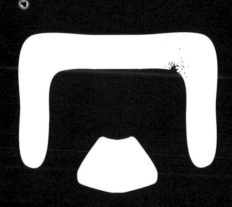

For the moustache lover on the go or the soirée-hosting tache connoisseur, here is a quick-fix to ensure you have a fine facial adornment for every occasion. Simply photocopy the following pages using thick paper, cut around the edges of the moustache and tape to a stick. Where there are beards, cut out separately and use a stick each for the moustache and goatee. *Et voilà*! Perfect party props!

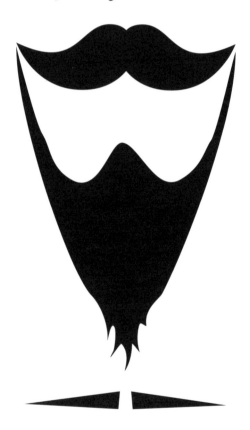

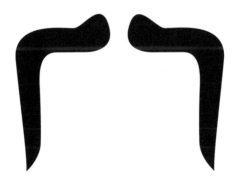

Party Props

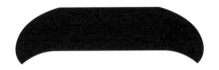

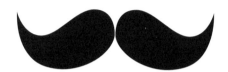

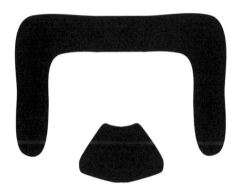

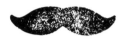

If you're interested in finding out more about our books, find us on Facebook at **SUMMERSDALE PUBLISHERS** and follow us on Twitter at **@SUMMERSDALE**.

WWW.SUMMERSDALE.COM